Organic Homemade Skin Care Recipes for Beginners:

Easy and Simple Instructions for Natural Remedies

Ginger Langley

Organic Homemade Skin Care Recipes for Beginners: Easy and Simple Instructions for Natural Remedies

Printed in the United States of America
April 2014

ISBN-13: 978-1497514676

ISBN-10: 1497514673

Table of Contents

Introduction

I am so pleased to present you with my personal collection of natural and homemade skin care recipes and remedies that I've been making and sharing with friends and family for the past ten years.

Please use these recipes and make adjustments as it suits your lifestyle and the people for whom you prepare these beauty treatments.

You will notice that I've purposely listed each remedy and skin care recipe on its own page. For me, it's easier to find those recipes when I need them.

If you like the natural formulations in this skin care book, you can let me know by writing a positive review on Amazon.com. I would be most grateful. Thank you.

All my best,

Ginger Langley

Chapter 1: Body Lotion Recipes Inspired By Mother Nature

There are many natural ingredients that help moisturize your skin. These include cocoa butter, almond oil, and coconut oil. When you use the recipes from this body lotion chapter, you will get beautiful skin at a fraction of the cost of store-bought lotions, AND you'll know that no harmful ingredients are finding their way into your body.

Shea Body Butter (For Dry, Normal, and Sensitive Skin)

This three-ingredient body butter is perfect for those searching for an organic solution to their moisturizing needs. The preparation of this homemade lotion is simple and easy.

Preparation Time:

Active time: 10 minutes
Processing time: 1 hour
Yield: 2 cups

Ingredients:

1 cup Shea Butter
1/2 cup Coconut Oil
1/2 cup Almond Oil

Storage Container: Sterilized glass container with a tight-fitting lid to hold the body butter lotion.

Directions:

Simply combine 1 cup of Shea butter and 1/2 cup of coconut oil in a double boiler. Melt the Shea butter and coconut oil, stirring frequently. When the mixture is melted, remove the top of the double boiler and place it on a heatproof surface.

Allow the mixture to cool for approximately 30 minutes. Once the body butter has cooled to room temperature, slowly stir in 1/2 cup almond oil.

Place mixture into a sterilized glass container, such as a small-sized canning jar with a screw-top, tight-fitting lid and then put the jar in the refrigerator. Keep the mixture in the refrigerator until the mixture starts to solidify. Once the mixture begins to solidify, beat the mixture with an electric mixer or an electric mixing stick until it resembles the texture of whipped butter.

Place the Shea body butter into a sterilized glass jar and use it after you take a shower for best results.

If you want to give your Shea body butter a different scent, simply add a few drops of an essential oil into the mixture when you whip it.

Lavender Vanilla Body Lotion (For all skin types)

This wonderful lotion takes only a short amount of time to create; however, you will be amazed at how great this lotion makes your skin feel. The lavender in this lotion creates a calming effect, which makes it a perfect go-to lotion for those stressful times in your life.

Preparation time: 30 minutes
Yield: 2 cups

Ingredients:

> 3 Tablespoons Organic Shea Butter
> 2 Tablespoons Coconut Oil
> 1/4 cup Lavender-Vanilla Infused Olive Oil*
> (Homemade recipe below.)

Storage Container: BPA-Free Plastic bottle with a squirt top and lid (like the mustard and ketchup bottles you'd take on a picnic).

NOTE: To make this lotion, you will either need to purchase lavender-vanilla infused olive oil, or you can make your own like I do. Just note that it takes about two months for the homemade version of infused oil to be ready. I'll give you my recipe below, if you'd like to make it yourself instead of buying it.

Directions:

Melt 3 tablespoons of organic Shea butter and 2 tablespoons of coconut oil in a heavy saucepan over low heat. Add in 1/4 cup vanilla-lavender infused olive oil. Stir until well blended.

Remove from heat and allow mixture to cool to room temperature. Then place the mixture in a lotion bottle.

Directions For Making Homemade Lavender-Vanilla Infused Olive Oil

Making a lavender-vanilla infused olive oil is an easy process. Simply add one cup of lavender blooms (from your own garden or from a local nursery) and one vanilla bean into a pint-sized canning-type glass jar with a lid. Then pour extra virgin olive oil over the blooms and vanilla bean, allowing the oil to cover the lavender and vanilla bean. Allow this mixture to develop by placing the jar in a cool dark location for two to four months. Shake the jar weekly (you might want to set a reminder to do this step) to help pull the scent out of the vanilla bean and the lavender blooms.

Once you have your vanilla-lavender infused olive oil, you are ready to begin making this fabulous lotion.

Summary

The recipes listed above have been inspired from natural ingredients known to help promote healing and restore moisture to your skin. Whip up a batch and begin allowing Mother Nature to heal your skin.

Chapter 2: Cold Cream That's Made With Natural Ingredients

My grandmother swore by her cold cream and used it religiously every night. She died when she was 85, but honestly, her skin always looked like a young woman's skin, because she used her own homemade natural remedies. I remember her skin feeling so soft that I just wanted to rub my face against hers. Believe it or not, my grandmother had very few wrinkles on her face. I know, some medical doctors would pipe up that it was her genetic makeup that gave her that smooth and flawless skin. But you and I both know that besides the environment and what we put into our bodies, a lot has to do with what we put on our skin.

Many years ago, I talked with her about how she made her natural and organic cold cream. When I began making these recipes for my own personal use, it wasn't until recently that I thought her little homemade recipes might need to be shared with other people, so they could achieve the same results that I have.

What follows are the recipes that she shared with me, and some that have been enhanced with my own additional ingredients. I hope you will enjoy them.

Chamomile-Infused Cold Cream

Chamomile tea is known to create a calming effect in your body as well as on your skin. Chamomile has been shown to soothe skin irritations and help prevent acne flare-ups. Additionally, chamomile is known to lighten age spots, which makes it a perfect addition to your cold cream.

Preparation Time: 45 minutes

Yield: 2 cups

Ingredients:

3 chamomile tea bags

1/4 cup distilled water

1/4 teaspoon Borax

1/2 cup almond oil

2 teaspoons beeswax

Additional Equipment and Storage Container

To make full use of this recipe, you will need a microwave, a blender, and a microwave-safe container.

Directions:

To make chamomile-infused cold cream, steep three chamomile tea bags in 1/4 cup distilled water. Allow the tea to steep 20 minutes to get its full benefits. Once the tea has cooled, you can begin making your cold cream.

Dissolve 1/4 teaspoon of Borax into your chamomile tea and set aside. Combine 1/2 cup almond oil and 2 tablespoons of beeswax in a heavy saucepan. Heat the almond oil and beeswax over low heat, stirring occasionally until the beeswax is melted.

In a small microwave-safe container, heat the Borax chamomile tea mixture for one minute. Place the almond oil and beeswax into a blender. Blend while slowly drizzling the Borax tea mixture into the blender. Blend until the mixture turns glossy white and is thick.

Pour the mixture into a pint-sized glass jar. Let cool to room temperature, and then seal the jar. Now, you're ready to use the cold cream.

Cold Cream with Tomato Toner

The following recipe combines the benefits of a cold cream with the benefits of a toner; thus, saving you a step when you remove your makeup at night.

Yield: 1 Cup

Ingredients:

2 tablespoons grated beeswax

1/4 cup extra virgin olive oil

1/4 cup extra virgin coconut oil

3 tablespoons tomato toner (homemade recipe follows)

A few drops of eucalyptus oil

Directions:

To make this cold cream, combine 2 tablespoons of grated beeswax with 1/4 cup extra virgin olive oil and 1/4 cup extra virgin coconut oil in a heavy saucepan. Heat this mixture over low heat until the beeswax melts and looks clear. Then add 3 tablespoons of tomato toner and a few drops of eucalyptus oil. Whip together until the mixture forms a rich cream that is similar to the look and consistency of a whipped topping.

Store this cold cream in a glass container or jar for easy accessibility and use.

Directions For Making Tomato Toner

Tomato toner contains vitamins A and C and is good for clearing acne and blackheads. It helps shrink pores and helps control oily skin. Use the pulp from an organic tomato and spread it on blackheads, acne, and blemishes on your skin like a mask to clear it up. (This isn't part of the recipe, but I thought you might want to know what to do with leftover tomato pulp.)

Cut about two inches of a cucumber and remove the skin with a peeler. Then juice, puree, or blend the cucumber so you just have the cucumber juice (approximately 3 tablespoons).

Using an organic tomato, cut off a few slices and mash it, using a blender, a juicer, or a tablespoon until you have about 3 tablespoons.

Combine the tomato juice with the cucumber juice in a cup or glass (quantities should equal about half of each juice). Then add 1 teaspoon of juice from an organic lime to the cucumber-tomato mixture. That's it. Now you have the tomato toner for the cold cream recipe.

Summary

Both of these cold cream recipes are sure to keep wrinkles at bay. The all natural ingredients you put on your face will ensure that your skin stays looking its best.

Chapter 3: A Natural and Organic Facial Mask

Women today have so many options of beauty treatments, it is impossible to keep track of what is in them and what they do. When you look at the ingredients, do you know what the chemicals are? I certainly don't, and I have been using beauty products for over a decade. In fact, I once heard a naturopath say that if you read the label of a health or beauty product and you don't understand the names of the ingredients, then don't buy the product.

Manufacturers try to blind us with science, and in most cases, it works. We end up buying a product, because it has some miraculous chemical in it we know nothing about.

Not only do we have no idea of what we are putting on our bodies, we also have to pay extortionate prices for the privilege of doing so. Thinking of it this way does tend to make us look a little bit silly, so to give control back to ourselves, why don't we use a natural skin care recipe? That way, we know exactly what is in it and the costs are low.

Using natural homemade skin care products also helps the environment by reducing the amount of chemicals big industry produces. If we all made our own homemade organic products, then there would be no need for animal testing, which is one of the hidden parts of the beauty industry.

Preparing and mixing up your own recipe is pretty simple, and if you have children or grandchildren, even they can do it. It also gives you great pleasure and it's even a fun experience if you do it with a few friends and make a night of it.

Natural and Organic Facial Cucumber Mask

This recipe is for a facial mask made from cucumber, which is well known for its skin helping properties, oatmeal for exfoliating, and honey for that gentle smoothness. You will not find anything more natural than this in the shops, and it is great for cleaning and moisturizing the skin.

Yield: 2 applications

Storage Container: Glass or plastic

Ingredients:

2 teaspoons plain oatmeal (already cooked)

1 teaspoon extra virgin olive oil

6 teaspoons of mashed or pureed cucumber

1 tablespoon organic honey

Directions:

In a bowl, combine all the ingredients. Then simply mix all these gently together until you have a nice smooth, but thick paste.

If the mixture appears to be too runny, add a little more oatmeal, but if you want it thinner, add a bit more olive oil. You can check the consistency by placing a small amount of the paste between your fingers, and if it feels OK to you, then it is ready for use.

You then just apply it as you would any face mask. Leave it on for about 10 to 15 minutes, and then rinse it off. First, use warm water to open the pours, and then use cold water to close up your pores.

Do this every day, and after a week you should notice a positive and radiant complexion staring back at you in the mirror.

Chapter 4: Natural Remedies for Controlling and Healing Acne

Mother Nature gives people many ways to actively combat acne. If you are trying to get rid of acne, use some of the recipes listed in this chapter.

Apple Cider Vinegar Toner To Combat Acne

Combine 1/4 cup of apple cider vinegar with 2 tablespoons of witch hazel, 1/2 cup of distilled water and 10 drops of tea tree oil. Place these ingredients in a glass bottle, apply the liquid to a cotton pad, and smooth it on your face daily after washing your face for best results.

Thyme Moisturizer to Help Control Acne

Combine equal parts of coconut oil and cocoa butter in a double boiler. Heat on a very low temperature until the cocoa butter is thoroughly melted. Allow the mixture to cool to room temperature. Then, beat with a handheld mixer until thoroughly blended. After the mixture is whipped into a lotion, slowly add 2 to 3 drops of thyme essential oil for each tablespoon of moisturizer.

Egg White Acne Mask

Before placing any mask on your face, you need to wash your face and moisturize it. The best way to moisturize your face before an egg white mask is to gently massage Vitamin E oil into your skin, and let it sit on your face for 30 minutes.

Next, beat an egg white until frothy. Apply the egg white to your face and allow it to cure on your face for 30 minutes. Finally, rinse your face with cold water and blot dry. Your face should feel sparkly clean.

Spot Treatment For Acne Using Aspirin

Aspirin is known to treat a variety of ailments, including acne. Because of the salicylic acid in aspirin, this spot treatment helps reduce swelling and redness caused by acne. To make this natural remedy, simply mash one uncoated aspirin with 4 drops of water. You can place the aspirin between two spoons to mash them. Mix this together and apply to your acne. Allow this mixture to sit on your acne for five minutes. Then, rinse off the solution.

This procedure can be repeated up to one week, using daily applications. After that time, you should be able to visibly seen the healing results.

Baking Soda Facial Wash

Baking soda is known to help combat acne due to its neutralizing properties. To make a facial wash, simply place a little baking soda in a small bowl and add enough water to make a paste. Gently coat your face with the mixture and massage the paste into your pores. Allow the mixture to remain on your face for ten minutes; then, rinse with cool water.

Summary

As this chapter has shown, there are many items you can find around your house to help you fight acne. The next time your skin flares up, you can whip up a batch of homemade acne treatments for beautiful skin.

Chapter 5: Now You Can Cure Those Ugly Stretch Marks Using Natural Ingredients

Stretch marks occur when your skin stretches beyond its elasticity levels. Stretch marks are essentially fine lined scars that show your skin was stretched beyond its ability to stretch. There are many things you can do to help diminish the look of these stretch marks.

Exercise

Exercise is one of the best ways to help your skin regain its elasticity. By exercising, your skin regains some of its firmness which helps diminish the appearance of stretch marks.

Foods

By including a variety of proteins into your diet along with foods rich in Vitamins C and E, you can help promote healing of damaged skin tissue. Additionally, foods that are rich in the mineral zinc have been shown to help prevent stretch marks. Finally, foods rich in Vitamin K help promote the healing of your skin.

Aloe Vera

Aloe Vera is known to help tighten and tone the skin. Aloe Vera also contains enzymes that are known to help promote healing to damaged tissues. To use this healing plant, simply massage the Aloe Vera pulp into your stretch marks every day when you get out of the shower.

Lavender Oil

Lavender oil has been known to help lessen the appearance of stretch marks. Lavender oil should be applied to stretch marks three times a day. As the lavender oil helps regrow new skin tissue, the stretch marks will gradually start fading.

Apricot Scrub

Apricot scrubs are made from a mixture of ground apricot pits and apricot juice. This scrub exfoliates dead cells and damaged skin tissue. The apricot helps to tone and firm the skin which helps stretch marks disappear over time.

Aromatic Oils

There are many aromatic oils that promote healing to the skin. These oils also help to tone the skin. Combine chamomile oil, sweet almond oil, avocado oil and jojoba oil with lavender oil to help prevent and diminish the appearance of stretch marks. A good ratio is 1:1, meaning that every oil you add to a mixture should consist of the same amount. For example, if you add 1 teaspoon of chamomile oil, then you would also add 1 teaspoon each of sweet almond oil, avocado, jojoba oil, and lavender oil.

Homemade Stretch Mark Butter

In a medium-sized saucepan, combine 1/2 cup cocoa butter with 2 tablespoons of wheat germ oil along with 2 teaspoons each of sesame seed oil, apricot kernel oil, and vitamin E oil. Finally, add 4 teaspoons of grated beeswax and mix it with the other ingredients already in your saucepan.

Cook this mixture over very low heat until all the ingredients have melted.

Remove the pan from the heat and add in 2 teaspoons of vanilla extract. Pour into small jars and allow to cool completely. Once cooled, cap each jar and use as needed. This recipe yields approximately one cup of stretch mark butter.

Summary

Mother Nature has many all-natural ingredients available to you for preventing and diminishing the appearance of stretch marks. Use the ingredients and recipes listed above to help avoid stretch marks.

Chapter 6: Natural Remedies For Rosacea

Rosacea is characterized by a flushed appearance to your face along with small bumps under the skin's surface. Finding natural ingredients to help combat rosacea is paramount to sufferers, because many of the chemicals found in traditional face washes actually worsen the appearance of rosacea.

In this chapter, you are provided with a number of natural remedies without chemicals or expensive ingredient costs that promise to provide solutions for your rosacea-related skin maladies.

Four Ingredient Rosacea Facial Wash

Yield: 1 pint

Ingredients:

1/4 cup castor oil

1/4 cup clover honey (local, if available)

1 teaspoon tea tree oil (any brand)

3/4 cup extra virgin olive oil (any brand)

Container:

1 pint-size glass jar with lid

Directions:

To make this simple facial wash, just combine the castor oil, honey, tea tree oil, and olive oil in a glass jar. Place the lid on the jar and vigorously shake it to incorporate the ingredients together.

To use the facial wash, shake the jar for approximately one minute. Splash warm water on your face. Then, pour about a nickel-sized amount into the palm of your hand. Gently massage the facial wash into your skin using a circular motion for two to three minutes. Rinse well using lukewarm water and pat dry with a natural cotton towel (if available). Follow with an all-natural toner and moisturizer.

Both castor oil and olive oil are humectants. This means that these oils help your skin retain more moisture. By basing your facial wash on humectants, you can increase the moisture in your facial wash.

Lack of moisture is one of the primary causes for rosacea outbreaks.

The honey in the facial wash has antibacterial and antimicrobial properties. Honey also cleanses the skin while adding an extra layer of moisture into your facial wash.

NOTE: For extra antibacterial and antimicrobial impact, use an organic honey produced from around your local area.

Finally, the tea tree oil is a natural antiseptic. It also has antifungal properties, which makes it perfect for anyone who suffers from rosacea and is seeking a healing remedy.

Chilled Chamomile Tea

Chamomile tea is known to lighten dark skin pigmentation, relieve stressed skin, and help heal broken capillaries. For best results, brew chamomile tea for twenty minutes and allow it to cool. Soak a clean washcloth in the solution and place over your face for ten minutes to help relieve rosacea symptoms.

Licorice Aloe Vera Honey Mask

To make this soothing mask, combine one teaspoon of honey with one teaspoon Aloe Vera gel. Then add in one tablespoon licorice powder and blend well. Apply this mask mixture to your face and allow it to penetrate and work its magic for at least 15 minutes. Wash the mask off using lukewarm water. Then pat dry with a cotton towel.

Summary

Nature provides many ingredients to help people who are suffering from rosacea. The recipes above will help you create an all-natural beauty routine for your rosacea.

Chapter 7: Natural Remedies for Making the Perfect Facial Moisturizer

Your kitchen holds the key to having beautiful soft skin. All you need is a few ingredients to create the perfect facial moisturizer. Below, you will find several recipes to help you prevent wrinkles while maintaining beautiful glowing skin.

Two-Ingredient Facial Moisturizer

This two-ingredient moisturizer has scents that remind you of a day spent languishing on the beach. To make this organic, all-natural moisturizer, you need only two ingredients—coconut oil and cocoa butter.

To make, simply place both the coconut oil and the cocoa butter in a small pan and heat on a very low temperature until the cocoa butter is melted. Once the mixture is melted, allow it to cool slightly before placing it in a sealed container (glass is preferred, but you can also use a BPA-free plastic container). Shake the mixture vigorously to incorporate the ingredients together. Let the mixture sit for five minutes and then shake it again.

Separate the moisturizer into small jars, so you can keep a small amount on your sink counter and keep the rest in the refrigerator to extend the shelf life of your moisturizer. I prefer to use the tiny glass canning jars that are about two ounces. For me, this is the perfect size, but depending upon how much you use your all-natural moisturizer, you might want to use a four-ounce glass jar. I've found that this moisturizer easily keeps in the refrigerator for 30 days, but hopefully, if you use it every day, or several times a day, it will only be refrigerated for two weeks.

  The moisturizer mixture may solidify during cooler temperatures. If this happens, then all you have to do is simply place some moisturizer on the palms of your hands and rub together to heat the mixture. The heat that is generated will warm up the moisturizer so that you can easily spread it on your face.

Aloe-Inspired Facial Moisturizer

In a small saucepan, combine 3/4 cup beeswax, 1/2 cup almond oil, and 1 tablespoon of cocoa butter. Allow this mixture to melt slowly over very low heat.

In a separate bowl, mix 1 teaspoon Vitamin E oil along with 10 drops of your favorite essential oil. (It doesn't matter which essential oil you choose; sometimes you might just like the fragrance and that's okay.) I buy essential oils when they are on sale, so you might want to check into that option, too.

Pour the melted beeswax, cocoa butter, and almond oil into a blender and allow to cool to room temperature. Do not skip this step or separation will occur!

Once cooled completely, blend these ingredients on low speed while slowly pouring the Aloe Vera mixture into the blender. Continue blending until the mixture has the look of a luxurious lotion. Scrape down the sides of the blender as needed.

Once the lotion has come together, pour the lotion into clean, sterilized jars. The contents in the jars will last approximately 6 weeks if kept refrigerated. By placing the lotion into small jars, you can keep all excess lotion refrigerated, while keeping one jar on your dressing table or in your bathroom for immediate use.

Summary

The lotions mentioned in this chapter use natural ingredients to moisturize your skin without containing any chemicals. These lotions allow you to thoroughly moisturize your skin without it feeling greasy. Remember to wash your face thoroughly before applying any type of moisturizer.

Chapter 8: Natural Remedies To Help Prevent Wrinkles Around Your Eyes

Mother Nature has many ingredients that you can use to help prevent wrinkles. The area around your eyes is susceptible to wrinkles, because the skin is very delicate. Because of this, many people want an anti-wrinkle eye cream that is gentle enough for their delicate skin, yet strong enough to fight crow's feet.

Vitamin E and Coconut Oil Eye Cream Recipe

There are many different eye cream recipes available that you can choose to use. One of the easiest to make can be created using only two ingredients. Simply combine Vitamin E oil and coconut oil in equal parts. Then gently pat on your eye area before bedtime. Vitamin E is known to help moisturize the skin; while coconut oil supports healing and tissue repair because of its antioxidant properties.

Turmeric, Lemon Juice and Honey Eye Cream Recipe

Another recipe using natural ingredients is to combine two teaspoons of honey, along with a little bit of turmeric and a couple of drops of lemon juice.

Take this mixture and massage it gently around your eyes. Let the mixture sit on your face for 15 minutes, then rinse and pat dry with a cotton towel.

The honey in the recipe is a natural humectant, which means it helps your face retain its natural moisture. The turmeric is used to help even out your skin making it perfect to help banish those dark circles under your eyes. Finally, the lemon juice is a natural way to help remove dead skin cells from your face.

The Easy-to-Make Eye Cream that Lasts a Month

The last recipe in this chapter combines several ingredients to make enough eye cream to last you about a month.

Simply place equal parts of jojoba oil, beeswax, and apricot kernel oil in a small saucepan. Slowly heat the mixture using low heat until the beeswax is just melted.

Remove the oils and liquid beeswax from the heat and whisk until combined.

In a separate saucepan, warm an equal amount of rose water. Once the rose water is heated, add two teaspoons of Borax powder to the rose water and stir until dissolved.

Place the oils and liquid beeswax in a small bowl that is sitting in an ice bath. Using a small whisk, beat the wax and oils, and then quickly add in the rose water Borax mixture. The eye cream will set very quickly using this technique.

Once the cream is totally cool, add two teaspoons of carrot-seed essential oil into the cream, folding gently. Then, place the completed cream in a small jar with a tight fitting lid. Yield is approximately one cup.

Summary

Any of the recipes listed in this chapter will help prevent wrinkles using only natural ingredients.

Chapter 9: All-Natural Eye Makeup Remover Recipes

When it comes to your eyes, nothing is as important as using quality ingredients you can trust. By using all natural ingredients, you can rest assured that nothing you put on your face is going to cause side effects. The eye makeup remover recipes in this chapter offer you several different all-natural ingredients and methods for you to try.

Witch Hazel Eye Makeup Remover

This simple recipe can be made using a variety of oils; however, I prefer to use extra virgin olive oil. It is less expensive, and I always have some in my pantry. To make this, simply grab a small glass jar or bottle and combine 4 tablespoons of witch hazel, 4 tablespoons of extra virgin olive oil, and 4 tablespoons of filtered water. Shake the container to ensure everything is mixed well. To use, soak a cotton ball in the eye makeup remover and gently swipe across your eyes. You will be amazed how quickly this works.

Non-Greasy Eye Makeup Remover that Removes Even Waterproof Mascara

This eye makeup remover contains castile soap; however, the amount is so tiny that it does not cause irritation to your eyes. This eye makeup remover can be made in a pint jar.

Simply place 1 cup of distilled water into your jar, then add 1/2 teaspoon liquid castile soap, and 1 teaspoon of extra virgin olive oil. Mix all ingredients by shaking the jar.

To use, simply dip a cotton ball in the solution and wipe across each eye to remove all traces of your eye makeup, including your waterproof mascara.

Two-Ingredient Miracle Eye Makeup Remover Recipe

This eye makeup remover is the easiest all-natural eye makeup remover available to anyone who loves to make homemade remedies. It contains only two ingredients. Both of these ingredients can be found in most households. If you do not have these ingredients, you can easily and conveniently pick them up at your local health food store or grocery store.

To make this recipe, simply combine equal parts of extra virgin olive oil and almond oil into a small glass jar or bottle and shake well.

To use, simply soak a cotton ball in the solution and wipe gently across your eyes to clean all traces of eye makeup from your face. Follow by rinsing your eye area with lukewarm water and pat dry with a cotton towel.

Summary

The all-natural eye makeup remover recipes in this chapter have several things in common, however, each recipe is a little different. The best thing about these formulas is they are made using all natural ingredients. By using easy-to-find and affordable natural ingredients, you can protect the fragile skin around your eyes while saving a ton of money.

Chapter 10: Facial Scrubs Inspired By Nature

When it comes to putting something on your skin, you most definitely want a facial scrub that's gentle and effective. When you use natural ingredients and make your own homemade facial scrubs yourself, you are ensured that you will not be putting chemicals on your face. The following recipes will help you create natural facial scrubs that give your skin that inner glow and radiance, while at the same time, keeping your skin healthy.

Baking Soda Facial Scrub

Baking soda is not only great for cooking, it is also great for your skin. The small particles found in baking soda are perfect for exfoliation. To make a baking soda scrub, simply mix 1/4 cup of baking soda with a small amount of water to make a paste. Then, apply the paste to your face and massage it in using a circular motion. Allow the baking soda paste to sit on your face for 15 minutes. Then, rinse your face with cool water and gently pat your face dry with a cotton towel.

Sweet Sugar Scrub

Granulated sugar is a natural exfoliate that can be found in almost any kitchen. To make a sweet sugar scrub, combine 1 teaspoon of granulated sugar with 1/2 teaspoon organic honey. Stir until both ingredients are mixed well. Then, add 1/2 teaspoon of lemon juice to the scrub mixture. The sugar helps to exfoliate dead skin cells from your face. The honey is a natural antioxidant. The lemon juice helps clarify the skin, making it a perfect facial scrub for everyone, but especially for men and women suffering from acne.

Caffeine-Inspired Facial Scrub

Coffee is one of the best exfoliators you can find, due to the particle size of ground coffee. Coffee contains anti-inflammatory properties along with collagen boosting caffeine.

To make this scrub, combine 1 tablespoon of ground coffee with 1 tablespoon of extra virgin olive oil. Apply this scrub using a circular motion. Then, gently buff off with a moistened washcloth. Finally, splash your face with cool water and pat dry. The extra virgin olive oil acts as a natural moisturizer allowing you to skip your moisturizer.

The Best Oatmeal Scrub

For ages, oatmeal has been known to provide soothing relief to irritated skin. Now, you can make a wonderful oatmeal scrub with only a few ingredients.

To make an oatmeal scrub, combine 1 tablespoon of dry, ground oatmeal, 1/4 teaspoon of salt, and 1 teaspoon of extra virgin olive oil. Blend these ingredients into a paste and apply to your skin using gentle circular motions. Allow the oatmeal scrub to sit on your face for 10 minutes; then, rinse with cool water and pat dry with a cotton towel.

Summary

All of the recipes listed in this chapter use natural ingredients. By using natural ingredients, you can not only save money, but you can protect your health from chemicals commonly found in commercially-sold facial scrubs.

Did You Like This Book?

It looks like you've made it all the way to the end of my book. I'm very happy you enjoyed it enough to get all the way through the recipes and health benefits. Hopefully, you've earmarked several recipes that you'll try today or this week.

If you liked the book, would you be open to leaving me an honest review? If you can take a minute, I'd really appreciate you writing a review on the Amazon website so others can discover how easy and healthy it is to use coconut milk in everyday recipes. It would really mean a lot to me.

Thank you!

Ginger Langley

About the Author

Ginger Langley lives in the Pacific Northwest, and she loves to cook and experiment with new healthy recipes.

Don't forget to check out these best-selling books, also by Ginger Langley:

Coconut Oil Cookbook: Quick and Easy Recipes for Busy People Who Want to Eat Healthy

Juicing Recipes for Weight Loss, Vitality and Health

Coconut Milk Recipes: 21 Quick & Easy Meals for Breakfast, Lunch, Dinner, and Dessert

Vitamin Water Recipes: Quick & Easy Homemade Vitamin Drinks Made From Fruits & Vegetables

Contact Me

If you have any questions for me, or if you have a story you'd like to share about how any of these natural skin care remedies improved your well-being, you can contact me here:

gingerlangley1@gmail.com

NOTES